I0421771

Talking Back to MS

How I Beat Multiple Sclerosis Using Low-Dose Naltrexone

Elizabeth J. Rhodes

www.TalkingBackToMS.com

Copyright © 2013 Elizabeth J. Rhodes

All rights reserved. No part of this publication may be reproduced, distributed, or transmitted in any form or by any means, including photocopying, recording, or other electronic or mechanical methods, without the prior written permission of the author and publisher, except as allowed by the Copyright Act of the United States 1976, as amended.

Published by The Virtual Wizard

www.TheVirtualWizard.com

Liability Disclaimer

This book is intended to serve only as a resource and educational guide. The author does not assume medical or legal responsibility of having the contents of this book considered as a prescription for anyone, nor shall the author in any event be held liable to any party for any direct, indirect, punitive, special, incidental or other consequential damages arising directly or indirectly from any use of this material. By reading this book, you assume all risks associated with using the advice given below, with a full understanding that you are solely responsible for anything that may occur as a result of putting this information into action in any way, and regardless of your interpretation of the advice.

The author and publisher of this book and accompanying materials have used their best efforts in preparing this book.

The author and publisher make no representation or warranties with respect to the accuracy, applicability, fitness, or completeness of the contents of this book.

Some of the names have been changed to protect identities.

Terms of Use

You are given a non-transferable, "personal use" license to this book. You cannot distribute it or share it with other individuals.

Also, there are no resale rights or private label rights granted when purchasing this document. In other words, it's for your own personal use only.

Dedications

Many thanks to my husband, Tom, who stood by me through all of the difficult challenges as well as the victories I experienced with this awful illness. For keeping a brave face so I wasn't scared, especially when helping me with my nightly injections, I appreciate you more than you will ever know.

To my sister, Eleanor, who has suffered with Multiple Sclerosis for almost 30 years, and has remained positive and strong, and has inspired me beyond measure.

I also want to thank someone I didn't have the pleasure of meeting before his demise in 2010, Dr. Bernard Bihari, who was responsible for discovering the effectiveness of Low-Dose Naltrexone on the immune system in his groundbreaking clinical trial of patients with HIV/AIDS, and subsequent findings in the treatment of MS. Without his research and diligence, I would probably be in a wheelchair today.

Acknowledgements

I want to thank everyone who helped me in the process of writing this, my first book. First of all, the many, many individuals who were diagnosed with Multiple Sclerosis who inspired me to tell my story in this manner. I am so happy to be able to help so many people to realize the same successes I have in my journey with this illness. You can join and support us at:

https://www.facebook.com/groups/TalkingBackToMS/

For doing such an amazing job with my book cover, I want to thank my graphic artist, Sanchita Dutta of BN Solution. You can contact her here at:

http://bnsolution.in/

I would also like to thank Jay Boyer and John S. Rhodes (no relation), without whose teachings, I would still be kicking around the idea of writing a book. And thanks for creating the author forum on Facebook, where I have formed many great friendships with fellow "authors" who have helped me tremendously, and squashed my publishing fears. Finally, thank you to my family who gave me the support and encouragement (and the "nudge") that made this book possible.

Introduction

Let me give it to you straight. I'm a no-nonsense kinda girl. That's the way this book is written. I'm not going to confuse you with a whole bunch of words you don't understand or can't pronounce. This is my story and I'm shooting straight from the hip.

Whether you have been newly diagnosed, or have had MS for years, this book has something of value to offer you.

I am not a medical professional, but I AM a person who has dealt with this disease for over 30 years, as I have a sister who was also diagnosed in the late 70s. Over these many years, it seems like everyone I meet has either personally been diagnosed, or has a friend or loved one who suffers from this condition. Once I tell people I have it, they give me a look of disbelief. By outward appearances, I don't *look* like I'm affected by Multiple Sclerosis.

One of the main reasons I chose to write this book is because I am asked almost daily what I am doing to stay so well and healthy-looking, and how I keep from relapsing.

I have given my "elevator speech" so many times over the years, I said to myself, "What the heck? Just write a book!" With this, I will be able to share my story with more people, and spread hope worldwide, instead of just in my local community.

I'm hoping that through reading about my challenges and victories you too can turn your life around. My mission is to help as many people as I can feel better and have a better quality of life.

Preface

I was brought up to question authority. If something doesn't seem quite right, I just flat out refuse it. Doctors are human beings just like you and me. They don't know everything, and are bound to make mistakes or bad decisions when it comes to healthcare. You are well within your rights to decline treatment if you don't want it. You do NOT have to ingest or inject chemicals into your body just because your doctor tells you to. Do your own research. Don't always rely solely on what your doctor says.

Doctors and pharmaceutical companies are not searching for cures. Think about it logically. If a cure is discovered for MS...or any other chronic or terminal illness, these people would go out of business! Yes, businesses exist in order to make money, and to ensure the stockholders and investors make *their* money. Cures don't make them money! Patients living better through chemicals *make them money*!

My intent through this book is to educate you through *my* story, and to encourage you to question and stand up to authority. It's your body. You should want what is best for it, not someone else's idea of what that may be.

Multiple Sclerosis is a very complex condition. No one, not even the so-called "experts", have a definitive idea of how it is acquired, nor do they have a concrete treatment to control it. All they have is a bunch of expensive, experimental chemical treatments to offer, with no idea as to whether or not they are going to help you. Let me emphasize "**experimental**". Even though they are "approved" by the FDA, no one knows for sure how they are going to affect you; and it's no guarantee that they are *good* for you.

What we DO know is these chemicals "invade" your body and deplete your immune system. They cause secondary illnesses, some of which may be irreversible. (Have you noticed all the commercial ads on television over the last few years about class-action lawsuits for people who have suffered from serious physical problems, and even death, as a result of some FDA-approved drug they were taking for anything from birth control to heart disease to urinary incontinence?)

Let me emphasize, take an active role in your own healthcare by doing your own research. Be cautious when being offered any treatment, and don't just accept it because your doctor told you to. They don't have all the answers, especially when it comes to Multiple Sclerosis.

It's YOUR body. Take the best care of it!

Chapter 1 – Wake Up!

Late October, 2006, the day started out like any other day. I woke up, took a shower, went to work, the whole bit. Nothing unusual or out of the ordinary took place this morning.

I came home early from work on this particular day, because Tom and I were going to the Santana in concert. This would be the first time we were seeing them live, so we were pretty excited. It being the end of October, I made sure I took a jacket with me, in case it got chilly later.

We drove to the venue without incident, but when we got there, the parking lot was jam packed. We had no choice but to park a good distance from the amphitheatre, so that meant some walking. I was wearing shoes with a bit of a heel on them, but I thought it would be no big deal walking in them since I had worn those same shoes to walk all over Pittsburgh with my sisters just a few months before. By the time we found our seats, I noticed my feet were aching, and appeared to have "fallen asleep". I attributed it to all the walking we had done before the concert, so I put it in the back of my mind...for the moment.

Throughout the concert, I noticed that the numbness in my feet was not going away. I thought maybe my feet were just cold, as we were sitting outside on a late October evening. I tapped my feet on the ground in an effort to "wake them up", but nothing happened. It just felt like I was pounding two lifeless objects at the ends of my legs. I felt no impact.

At first I didn't say anything to Tom, but he finally asked me why I kept slapping my feet on the ground. So, I told him they were numb, and attributed it to all the walking we had done, and the fact that I was wearing heels. Although I didn't admit it at the time, I was a little worried.

When the show was over, we left our seats and began our long trek back to the car. My feet were still feeling numb, but didn't say another word about it.

Chapter 2 – The Breakdown

Three days later, panic set in. I woke up numb from the waist down. From just below my rib cage all the way down to my toes...completely numb. I was able to get up and walk around, and to look at me, you would have never known anything was wrong. When I got up to use the bathroom, I freaked out. I couldn't feel myself pee! I knew I was peeing! I could hear it! But, I could not feel a thing...sensation, temperature, nothing! I started to cry. I called out to Tom to come the bathroom right away, and told him what was happening. What *was* happening? Something serious was going on; something that would change my life forever.

We decided we were going to see Dr. Ashby, my physician for the last seven years, and the only doctor I trusted. He didn't accept my new insurance, (I had recently changed insurance carriers, but I hadn't bothered to see the new doctor, because I was hardly ever in need of medical treatment) but I didn't care. Dr. Ashby had become like a brother to me, and I didn't want to talk to anyone else about this.

I gave Tom my boss' cell phone number, and he called to explain I would not be in to work. I proceeded to get dressed so we could race over to Dr. Ashby's.

When we arrived, we went straight over to the check-in assistant, and explained what was happening. Even though I had no appointment, they took me in right away.

Within minutes, Dr. Ashby came into the exam room, holding my chart. He asked a bunch of questions, as he ran instruments up and down my bare legs. I felt absolutely nothing. He poked various areas of my legs and torso with a very sharp object. Still nothing. He even pulled out a tuning fork and held it against my ankle. While I could kinda feel the sensation of vibration, I couldn't feel the coldness of the steel on my foot. I was getting more scared by the minute.

I told him that my sister, who is eleven years older than me, has had Multiple Sclerosis (See Glossary) for many years, and reasoned that I thought maybe that is what's going on with me. He appeared to be genuinely scared, but told me he doubted it was MS. He excused himself from the room, and promised to be back in a few minutes.

After he left the room, I leaned over the exam table and just bawled my eyes out. "I think I have MS, Tom! I think I have MS." I just kept repeating that over and over and over, crying the whole time. Tom attempted to calm me down, assuring me that Dr. Ashby was going to figure out what was going on with me and get me the help I needed.

I just kept crying, all the while thinking of how my sister, who was only 52 years old, was no longer able to walk on her own, and got around primarily with the use of a motorized scooter.

A few minutes later, Dr. Ashby returned and advised us that he thought I had a condition called "Cauda Equina Syndrome". He went on to explain that this is a serious neurologic condition where there is an acute loss of function of the lumbar plexus (See Glossary). Any compression of this region may disable the nerves. He asked me if I had ever fallen on my tailbone or had any car accidents with significant trauma to that area, to which I answered "No, I haven't".

He said he wanted me to get an MRI (See Glossary) right away. Now, I was even more scared. I never heard of this condition.

Dr. Ashby's nurse gave us the necessary paperwork, and we rushed to the Magnetic Resonance Imaging Center a few miles away. There appeared to be no one in the waiting room, so I was relieved. I was hoping we could get this over with in a hurry and get some answers as to what was going on.

Through sobs and stutters, I attempted to explain to the receptionist that we had just come from Dr. Ashby's office, what he thought was happening, and handed her the paperwork. She went into the back of the office for a few minutes and came back to the front desk to inform us they could not perform the MRI on me, because the ordering physician was not my primary care physician. Therefore, I would have to pay for the procedure out of pocket. She explained that I needed to get an order from my primary care physician of record and come back. Once I had done that, they would be able to do the scans.

We begged them to please make an exception, as I had not even been to see the new primary care physician yet, never even met him, and that the only reason we went to Dr. Ashby is because he has my entire medical history. "Sorry," she said, "we can't make any exceptions." I was so desperate to get answers.

How disappointing. My life was falling apart, I couldn't think straight, I was panicked, and scared, and confused, and I couldn't hold it together. I couldn't do anything except cry. I was so scared and worried, I just wanted to get this MRI over with so I could get answers and get on with fixing me.

With paperwork in hand, we trekked back up the highway to visit this new doctor, Dr. Bella, who I had never even met. Upon arriving there, we walked into a waiting room full of people. I started to panic again, because I was growing very impatient. I found an empty wall, leaned against it, slid all the way down to the floor, put my head in my hands and cried.

I consider myself to be a very strong person, but this situation was breaking me down to my very core. I just wanted to get answers so I could start feeling better right away, and it seemed like I just kept hitting what I considered "road blocks" at every turn.

While I sat against the wall in the waiting area having an apparent nervous breakdown, Tom went to the receptionist's window and explained my situation, quietly pleading with her that someone see me right away. A short time later, one of the medical staff came out into the waiting room and offered me some water. She tried asking me some questions, but I couldn't even speak.

I imagine I was disturbing all of the other patients waiting to be seen by the doctor, because they took me into an exam room within minutes.

As soon as I walked through the door, I found an empty corner and again sat on the floor and sobbed uncontrollably. When the doctor came into the room, Tom did all the talking. I couldn't even move, let alone speak. With Tom's help, the doctor urged me to get up off the cold, hard floor and sit on the examination table, where the doctor could break out his instruments and poke me. Through my sobs and hiccups, I told the doctor I felt nothing. The doctor basically called me psychotic in so many words and left the room.

This made me a little irate. So, when the doctor returned to the room, I pretty much yelled at him, called him uncaring and unfeeling, and a few other choice words I don't care to mention here. What kind of a doctor verbally insults someone when they are having a crisis?

I suppose I struck a nerve with *him*...one that *he* could actually feel, because he abruptly left the room and sent in one of his staff members.

The woman calmly sat me down and explained that I needed to go to the hospital down the street. She told me she had already called them, and they were expecting me. She went on to inform me they were going to admit me, and run a slew of tests and x-rays in an effort to find out what exactly is going on with me. With this news, I calmed down quite a bit. Finally, someone is going to take some tests and get to the bottom of my dilemma.

I hated hospitals, but even though I didn't want to be admitted, I breathed a huge sigh of relief. At least there they would be able to run all the tests they wanted, and I wouldn't have to run from doctor to doctor trying to get answers.

So, I tried to calm down and convince myself that this was going to be a positive experience, and that the staff at the hospital was going to take good care of me.

With all of this going on, still, in the back of my mind, I had settled on my self-diagnosis of Multiple Sclerosis.

Chapter 3 – Ah! So That's What That Was!

I always had this gnawing fear that I would end up with Multiple Sclerosis, just like my sister had many years ago. She began having symptoms sometime in the mid-80s, and almost thirty years later, she has lost complete control over the use of her legs. I had witnessed her slow deterioration over these many years, and prayed that would never happen to me.

Well, I guess as the saying goes, "What you think about you bring about" is true, because I thought about it all the time, full of dread that I would find myself in her same situation.

Now, here I was, 41 years old, having symptoms of what I believed to be Multiple Sclerosis.

I tried to reason with myself…"It can't be…two siblings from the same family?" It didn't seem possible, but, then again, there *are* nine of us kids. So, I guess odds are in favor of it happening. This is the rationalization that took place in my mind while I waited to be taken into my hospital room.

As the minutes ticked by, crazy memories began flooding at me. I was remembering the strange physical sensations and weird feelings that I had experienced over the years, and how I'd just dismissed them and didn't have them investigated. One memory, dating all the way back to elementary school, after I had taken my turn to run in a relay race, I sat down on the floor, and my foot started "thumping" uncontrollably. This lasted for over a minute, as I recall, and I tried to hide it from the other students by curling my legs up under me. You could visibly see my foot jumping up and down as if it were dribbling a basketball.

In my late teens, I stopped running completely, because it seemed like my ankle would "lock up" every time I attempted running, and I would either lose my step, or fall flat on my face. I got to a point where I just started telling everyone I had "weak ankles". Through my experiences with MS, I now know this is called Clonus. (See Glossary)

Another incident I recall from my teenage years, I had a cold sensation in my lumbar region and down my leg whenever I would move my body or my head a certain way. I told my mother about it, but she brushed it off; said I probably just slept in a weird position. It came and went several times over the years, without being investigated or treated. I now know there is a name for this, Lhermitte's Sign. (See Glossary)

In my early thirties, I recall times where, after taking walks during my lunch break, I noticed my legs were tingling. It felt like thousands of tiny insects were running all over them, and it would last for hours. I just attributed it to the fact that maybe I didn't exercise enough, and my blood vessels were just letting me know they were alive. Again, I didn't tell anyone, nor did I have it investigated.

There were other times when I would experience my feet falling asleep, but it would only last an hour or so...never days and days and days, like my current "attack". I would just dismiss it, thinking the cold, uncarpeted floor under my desk was the cause, so I invested in a portable heater.

Most recently, I want to say within the two months or so before my numbness "attack", on several occasions, I experienced a problem with my right eye going in and out of focus. This was a big problem for me, because at that time I was working as a Technical Writer at the time, and was studying for my Bachelor's degree. I estimate I was using the computer at least 12 hours a day. But, this problem went away just as quickly as it appeared. I later found out this eye condition is called Optic Neuritis, (See Glossary) and is one of the many symptoms experienced by people with Multiple Sclerosis.

Also of note during this time, Tom and I joined a local gym. A couple of my girlfriends and I started attending some of the classes offered there, including strength training with bungee cords. Part of this training required balancing, and I found myself unable to perform this simple thing. Also, I couldn't do as many reps as all the other ladies in the class, and I got fatigued very easily. In addition, at least once during a class I had sit down because I became quickly overheated and almost passed out. What the heck was going on??? These were simple exercises!!! Everyone told me I turned beet red, and a couple of them brought me bottles of cold water. I just dismissed it, attributing it to the fact that I had not worked out in many years, and was just really out of shape. Once again, I didn't mention it to Tom, and didn't visit the doctor to investigate.

In addition to all of my *real* symptoms, I also remember having recurring dreams over the years where I was walking up a hill and my legs didn't want to move. It was as if I were walking in wet cement. Was my brain trying to tell me something??? A premonition of things to come??? Perhaps. A foretelling of my future??? Interesting. (So, can I please have the dream where I am winning millions of dollars in the Lottery???)

I tried to think positive thoughts, but now while sitting in the hospital, waiting to be poked and prodded, and have "pictures" taken, all of these memories of past "signs" and symptoms came flooding at me. I had convinced myself that I had Multiple Sclerosis; and based on all of these memories from the past, I figured I must have had it for many years before; but time and time again, just dismissed my symptoms.

Chapter 4 – The Wait Begins

After racing over to the hospital, I waited for what seemed like an eternity for someone to take me to a room. I hated being in the hospital. It's so cold and lonely, especially when you don't know what to expect, and you're panicked out of your mind because your body is going haywire.

And even though Dr. Bella had acted like a jerk, admitting me to the hospital seemed like the best decision toward figuring out what was going on with my body.

Thankfully, all of the staff members I encountered at the hospital were very accommodating and overly courteous. That was just what I needed, after having my mini nervous breakdown earlier in the day.

A hospital staff aide finally came to take me to my room, and gave me some lovely designer duds to wear, along with those great slip- resistant socks with the tire treads on the bottom.

After I changed, and snuggled myself into my bed, the nurse's aide came into the room to get my vital signs, weight, etc. (It's very cool; you don't even have to get out of bed for them to check your weight. It's built right into the bed! Genius!) To my surprise, he was a young kid. If I had to guess, I would say he was about 19 or 20 years old. He looked very nervous, so I asked a few questions of him to calm *his* nerves. Imagine??? *Me* calming *his* nerves??? Through my mini interrogation, I discovered this was his very first week on the job.

He asked me a few questions, one of them being, "Do you need a bedpan"? "For what?" I asked. He glanced at my chart with a puzzled look on his face, and said, "You're numb from the waist down. Did you walk in here all by yourself?" To which I answered, "Yup."

This poor kid just didn't know what he was in for having me as a patient. So, I made light of it, and joked with him a bit about considering himself lucky that he wasn't going to have to give me a sponge bath! Of course, he turned red, but my joking did seem to ease his nerves a bit.

Not long after my nurse's aide, Todd, left the room, a nurse came in, wrote her name on the white board in front of me, and introduced herself. She was the evening shift nurse. (Holy crap! It was late afternoon already???) She asked a few questions, and explained she would be back shortly to take me down to Radiology to get some MRIs. Yay! MRIs. I had never had any of those before, and I wasn't sure what to expect. All I know is what other people told me about their experiences with MRIs. They said they hated it because they became very claustrophobic. Great! Now I really needed something to calm my panic.

Chapter 5 – Say Cheese!

So, into the wheelchair I go, off to Radiology. They said it was going to take a few hours to perform all of the MRIs the doctor had ordered, so Tom went home to get me a few essentials for my hospital stay.

Just as the other staff I had encountered had been, the MRI technicians were very nice and accommodating. I had tons of questions to ask about the whole process, and they answered every single one. This eased my mind quite a bit.

They asked me what brought me into the hospital today, and I told them about my numbness and how scared I was. They were very empathetic and understanding, and asked me if I needed help getting out of the wheelchair to walk over to the MRI machine. (Hmmm, apparently, when you're numb from the waist down, people automatically assume that means you are paralyzed, as well. Interesting.)

They explained how many different views they were going to take of my brain and my spine, and that I would be in that machine for a few hours. At some point, they went on to tell me, before the end of the "pictures", they were going to have to inject me with some Gadolinium (See Glossary), which is something that makes any scar tissue, also known as "lesions" (See Glossary) in your brain light up like a Christmas tree! This was done to show contrast to better find any "active disease".

Note to readers: Prepare yourselves. Anyone who has never had an MRI before, the sound is deafening! Ask them to give you headphones or ear plugs or something. I just wanted nothing more than to get the heck out of there.

Chapter 6 – And the Winner Is…

After a long, lonely week in the hospital, I was still no closer to having an answer to my health problems. I was getting kind of used to being in the hospital at this point, though. Every morning, one of the nurses would come in and take a few tubes of blood from me. I would get wheeled down to Radiology for yet another MRI. The nurses and I were also becoming "friends". They would share their smoothies with me, and let me "hang out" with them near the nurse's station outside of my room at night when I couldn't sleep. I was trying to stay positive, but I was absolutely exhausted and completely freaked out because I didn't know what was happening to me. But, I put on a good show and tried to act brave.

During this time, as if being in the hospital with my body betraying me weren't enough, my husband was let go from his job, because he wanted to spend time with me so I wasn't alone and lonely all day. (I don't understand this. It's not like the company was paying him a salary. They weren't paying for his benefits. He was working on commission, and wasn't paid until he sold a product. Baffling.)

I lay there in bed, day after day, talking to Tom, speculating about what the MRIs were going to show. We talked about how earlier in the week, Dr. Bella went over all of the blood tests with me, and they had found nothing. They tested for HIV, Lupus, Lyme Disease, all forms of Hepatitis, and a whole host of other diseases...all the results came back negative. So all we were waiting for was the results from the MRI scans. I was still convinced I was facing a diagnosis of Multiple Sclerosis.

Two different Neurologists (See Glossary) came in to see me several times during my hospital stay...Dr. Zoppa and Dr. Calderon. They asked a bunch of the same questions all the other doctors and nurses asked me since my problem began. They also ran their pointy instruments up and down my legs, just as the others had. In addition, they had me walk to the wall and straight back to them, balance and touch my nose with my eyes closed, and a few other neurological tests.

They would always leave the room without explanation, but I could hear them in the hallway, dictating their findings, and consulting with other doctors. Unfortunately, their voices were muffled, and I couldn't quite make out what they were saying. I was impatient, and I wanted answers, dammit!

So on this, my sixth day in the hospital Dr. Zoppa entered my room, just as he had for the previous four days, this time for the purpose of discussing my MRI scans. With a look of concern on his face, he flat out said, "Mrs. Rhodes, you have a hole in your brain."

WHAT!!! I wanted to scream!! What does that even mean? A big 'ol chunk of my brain is missing??? What kind of bedside manner was this?

I imagine the horrified look on my face must have scared him too, because he immediately began to back-pedal. "It is inconclusive", he said, "but based on your MRIs, it looks like you have Multiple Sclerosis." He went on to explain that he was going to perform a spinal tap to get a more conclusive "diagnosis".

He started to tell us that MS is not the "death sentence" it was thought to be years ago. He explained there were now many "promising" new treatment options formulated to suppress the disease progression, where previously there were *none*. This made me feel a little bit better, but I was still upset about his news delivery.

He went on to advise that he wanted me to get on a course of steroids (See Glossary) right away. He talked about the benefits, as well as the downsides, and told me to think about it. In basic terms, the steroids would help my symptoms to subside, but at the same time, they would strip my immune system, leaving me vulnerable to infection. As he was walking out the room, he told my husband and me to discuss it, and promised to return in a bit to perform the spinal tap.

The instant he left the room, I cried. I just completely lost it. Why in the world was this happening to me? Even though I had privately given myself the MS diagnosis, the reality of the words coming from his mouth freaked me out. Why was my body betraying me? I lived clean my whole life!! Didn't do any hard-core recreational drugs and didn't smoke. I wasn't an alcoholic by any stretch of the imagination. This just wasn't fair at all!

I immediately thought again about my sister, and pictured her in that scooter. This cannot happen in my life! I'm too young and have too many things I want to do! I don't want to end up not being able to walk for the rest of my life! "I'm going to live for another 50 years", I told myself. I will absolutely die if I have to spend 50 years in a wheelchair!!!

A few minutes later, an aide came into the room and placed a basin full of supplies in the chair at the foot of my bed. Without explanation, she left the room just as suddenly as she entered. I peeked over and saw a package that read, "Lumbar Puncture" (See Glossary). ACK! The thing I dreaded the most! Although I didn't want anyone messing around with my spine, Tom and I talked about it, and we agreed it was probably necessary as we were searching for answers.

Dr. Zoppa came back a short time later with a nurse and started scrubbing up for this procedure. I was deathly afraid of someone sticking a long needle into my spine and extracting fluid. I explained this to the doctor, so he ran through the whole process with us, step by step.

The procedure seemed to last forever! I was balled up on the edge of the bed with my knees in my chest, my arms tightly hugging around them, while Dr. Zoppa manipulated that needle into one of the spaces between my vertebrae, and extracted several small tubes of spinal fluid. (In reality, it only lasted about ten minutes, tops!)

When he was finished, the nurse cleaned off my back, applied a bandage helped me to lie down. I glanced at Dr. Zoppa, who was sweating profusely. His shirt was soaked through. I don't know if it was from nervousness or what, but it was over, and I was relieved...not only because it was over, but because the doctor had informed us that once I got the spinal tap, I didn't have to get another one!

The back pain during the procedure was very minimal, but the headache I suffered afterward was very intense. The doctor advised that I had to lie still for at least a couple of hours after the procedure. After that time, he advised, I would be able to go home.

As I lay there in bed, fighting off a headache, Tom and I discussed all the treatment options after the doctor left the room. We decided to *not* go down the road of steroids, as I didn't want to put my body through the depleted immune system crap.

When the doctor returned we gave him our decision about the steroids. He instructed me to come to his office the following week, and reminded me about the treatment options.

The nurse brought me the doctor's orders, and I happily signed my release papers. After a week in the hospital, I was anxious for a change of scenery.

All I could do for the next two weeks; however, was lay down, because I had a residual headache from the spinal tap. Needless to say, I had to file for FMLA (See Glossary) through work, so I didn't run the risk of losing my job. This required many telephone calls, and filling out a ton of paperwork. The whole process was a chore for me, because I was so depressed and experiencing the worst headache of my life. I had absolutely no ambition to do anything whatsoever. It was painful just opening my eyes. Thanks spinal tap.

But, at least I had a diagnosis.

Chapter 7 – You're Fired!

You know when you sometimes just have a feeling in your gut about something? You can't quite put your finger on it, but you have some doubts looming in your head? This is how I felt about Dr. Zoppa. When he came into the hospital room and told me I had a hole in my head, I thought, "What a jerk!" What kind of bedside manner is this? He's supposed to be helping me, not making me feel worse!

As it turns out, my feelings were completely justified the day of my post-hospital visit. When I walked into the practice he shared with Dr. Calderon, I started to have a panic attack. As soon as I sat down in the waiting room, I looked on the wall at all the Diplomas and Degrees. One thing blared out at me as if I had just hit my thumb with a hammer. (By the way, I have done this before, and I don't recommend it. OUCH!) All of the credentials that hung on the walls of this waiting room had one common theme. Dr. Zoppa and his colleagues were all only just barely a year out of medical school. What's more, the "managing" physician, who had been in practice for over twenty years, had just passed away in a car accident. (Yes, they had this newspaper article of the incident displayed on the wall, too.)

All I wanted to do was get out of there! But, there were no other neurologists in the area who accepted my insurance. So, I thought to myself, "I'm stuck with these guys who are barely out of medical school." No wonder Dr. Zoppa had such a hard time performing that spinal tap! It was probably the first one he ever performed! That kind of scared me.

But, I calmed down by reasoning to myself that maybe these doctors had some new tricks up their sleeves that the older docs don't know about. So, I gave them the benefit of the doubt.

Well, Dr. Zoppa, who specifically told me to come and see him a week after I got out of the hospital, was not there. Turns out, he was on vacation out of the country. So, I got saddled with Dr. Calderon, a doctor I had only met one time! Brilliant! Here comes the anxiety again.

I waited for a short time for Dr. Calderon to come into the examination room. He had my spinal tap results, and explained to me they were positive for the markers, known as "Oligoclonal Bands" (See Glossary) that usually show up for people who have MS.

He encouraged me to think about getting on a treatment right away. I told him I would think about it, and that I had to do some research into the approved MS drugs before I made my decision.

After leaving there, I still felt very uncomfortable about the lack of practical "experience" the doctors had. In addition, I was still freaked out about the "hole in the brain" thing. I decided I was going to search for a different Neurologist.

And the hits just keep on coming. During this same time period, I received a letter in the mail from Dr. Bella's office. The doctor "fired" me as a patient, because, as he put it, I was "very unstable and irate". Thanks for kicking me when I'm down. So now, on top of all the other stress I was dealing with, I had to find a new primary care physician. Maybe this was a blessing in disguise, because this guy hardly spoke any English...well, not that I could understand anyway. And, he didn't take very good care of me while I was in the hospital. (That's another story for another book.)

Chapter 8 – Doctor's Orders

As soon as I got back home from Dr. Zoppa's/ Dr. Calderon's office, I logged onto the computer in an attempt to find a different, experienced Neurologist. I had to perform a wide area-search, but finally found one. He was 30 miles away, but he accepted my insurance.

I did some research on this guy, and found out he had been practicing for 20+ years. I found a few websites with "health grades" to further my research of this doctor. In addition, I asked around to some folks in the medical industry who assured me he was top-notch. So, it was settled. I was going to make an appointment with Dr. McRae.

A few days later, I had my first appointment with Dr. McRae. He asked a lot of questions, looked at my MRIs that were taken at the hospital, and did a bunch of neurological tests for strength and balance.

As we were wrapping up the appointment, Dr. McRae handed me a kit for one of the "promising" new-fangled injectable drugs (Also referred to as "CRAB" drugs – See Glossary) that are specifically formulated to suppress the MS symptoms. The doctor instructed me to read all of the contents thoroughly. I was also given the telephone number to call a nurse who would come to my house to teach me how to give myself the injections. There was something else I had to order, and Auto-Injector pen (See Glossary), to assist me in giving myself the shots.

I walked out of this appointment with an order for a new round of MRIs, at a facility that Dr. McRae preferred, as well as a follow-up appointment which would include Evoked Potentials Tests (See Glossary), and Nerve Conduction Tests (See Glossary).

Figuring Dr. McRae must know best, being that he had so many years of medical school and in practice experience and all...with no questions asked, I did as the doctor instructed.

Chapter 9 – My New Life

I gave myself my first injection after dinner on Thanksgiving Day, 2006. I cried the whole time.

After a few weeks of daily injections, I decided I couldn't handle it. I was feeling sick and weak every day. I wasn't able to eat. I was also having bizarre, terrifying nightmares. In addition, my arms and hands were beginning to feel the same numb sensations I was experiencing in my torso, legs and feet. All I wanted to do was sleep, but that was an impossibility, because I was still working a full-time job, and going to school for my Master's Degree.

I made another appointment to see Dr. McRae to discuss the possibility of trying a different treatment.

Because of my failed attempt with the first drug, I had done some additional research on these "promising" MS treatments. During this visit with Dr. McRae, we talked about the other available options, and decided on a different injectable medication, because from everything I read, it seemed like the least "harmful" of all the other ones. The main selling points were that the shots were only three times a week and they were given just under the skin. If this didn't work, I was going to be forced to get drugs through infusion therapy. (See Glossary)

I hated it! I cried every single time I had to give myself that shot. I did all the research, and I knew all the associated risks; but, the doctor said it showed "promise". He said he had a lot of patients who realized very favorable results, so I tried to be optimistic and continued with the treatment.

Two months into this treatment I was forced to quit graduate school, because I was having a hard time concentrating. Also, holding a pen and taking notes was becoming a difficult chore, and my handwriting was becoming unreadable.

Although the numbness in my hips, legs, and feet was diminishing, I had another terrifying symptom, called the "MS Hug" (See Glossary). I am told not everyone with MS experiences it, but to give you an idea of what I was going through, it felt like my entire ribcage and chest was wrapped up very tightly, and constantly being squeezed tighter and tighter. I felt like I couldn't breathe. (I imagine this is what it feels like to be held captive by a boa constrictor.)

I watched my health continue to deteriorate, throughout the long four months of torture I endured with these "promising" new shots. The numbness I was experiencing just moved from one region of my body to another, without ever completely going away. In addition to the growing list of other symptoms, I developed bladder weakness and incontinence. The urinary urgency was sometimes so intense I could not make it to the bathroom. This was extremely embarrassing, as I was still working a full-time job!

My right leg was also in a continuous state of spasticity (See Glossary), and I had very little control over the movements of my right foot. Because of this, I couldn't pick my foot up off the floor, so it kind of just dragged behind me when I walked (more like "limped"). Through additional research, I found out this is commonly known in MS circles as "foot drop". (See Glossary) I had to buy several pairs of flat shoes, because I was unable to wear my beloved high heels anymore. During this time, Tom and I started talking about either buying a cane or asking around about used walkers.

Another terrifying symptom I discovered was that the hot water I normally used when taking a shower or washing dishes was now feeling like it was scalding my skin. And, handling ice cubes was excruciatingly cold. Even if it was only for a few seconds, I could hardly hold them. I later found out that this is caused by the impaired ability of the damaged nerves, known as "demyelinated" nerves (see Glossary) to properly conduct the electrical impulses to the brain.

I told Dr. McRae about these additional symptoms and problems, but he assured me this was "normal" with MS, and instructed me to continue with the injections. He also tacked on a prescription for a course of steroids, which he claimed should provide some symptom relief. At this point, I was desperate to feel better, so I agreed.

Without coming right out and saying it, Dr. McRae also alluded to us that based on how quickly my health was declining I was probably going to be in a wheelchair inside of two years. Needless to say, I felt as if I had just been handed a death sentence.

Based on this news, I started doing research on how to go about filing for Disability. In doing so, I found an interesting website that outlined the different "types" or "stages" of MS (see Glossary) as well as a chart called the "Expanded Disability Status Scale" or "EDSS" (See Glossary)

Chapter 10 – Denial

This was all happening way too fast. The medicine was supposed to be helping me get better, but I was getting worse. It seemed like every morning when I woke up I was faced with a new symptom. I was so depressed and felt so sorry for myself; I started preparing myself for the worst.

I made an appointment to see my "new" primary care physician, so I could get something for the continued panic attacks. In addition to anti-depressants, I started taking an anti-anxiety medication on a daily basis, thanks to Dr. Rutledge's handy little prescription pad. He also ordered a complete physical, and blood tests to check my liver function, because I told him about these injections I was taking.

I was so deep in that depression hole I didn't even tell my family what was going on. For some reason, somewhere deep down inside, I felt ashamed. I didn't want to worry anyone, least of all my father, who was suffering with his own health problems at that time. I already had one sister with MS; they didn't need to worry about me, too. I also stopped talking to all of my friends; I didn't' go out, and didn't accept phone calls. I went to the office and back home. That's it. Nowhere else.

Chapter 11 – Searching For a Miracle

While sitting at my desk at work one day, crying quietly to myself because my legs were so weak and shaky I couldn't get out of my chair to walk to the bathroom; I started doing an Internet search using my symptoms as keywords. I quickly scanned through the descriptions under the search results, and could not believe what I was seeing. Some little blurb someone wrote about a "miracle" drug that cured their MS! I clicked on the link to get more details.

It ended up being a message board where people diagnosed with MS visited to write about their experiences, and commiserate. I scrolled down the page through all of the posts, desperate to find the one I saw from the search results. Finally, after a few minutes, there it was! A woman who was diagnosed with MS several years earlier was describing this oral medication she was taking that completely cleared up all of her symptoms. She called this drug "LDN" (See Glossary). This surprised me, because I had never heard of this drug, and believe me, I had done a TON of research since my diagnosis! She described this drug as being "non-toxic" (See Glossary) and having "virtually no side effects". After seeing this, I had to do some more digging.

I opened up a new window and began to search for "LDN for Multiple Sclerosis". When the results came back, I couldn't believe my eyes! There was article upon article upon article, website after website, describing this LDN, or Low-Dose Naltrexone, and its benefits for people with MS and a whole host of other chronic illnesses. Why had I never heard of this before? Why didn't my doctor tell me about this treatment? No shots! No side effects! I felt betrayed and cheated!

The more reading I did, the more I thought, "This must be a hoax!" In my reasoning, there was just *no way* this "miracle" drug existed, yet my doctor had me giving myself these painful injections. Not only that, I wasn't getting any better. If anything, I was actually getting worse. Surely, if this was real, my doctor would have prescribed it for me.

I just knew this had to be a cruel joke someone was perpetuating on the Internet, and I wanted to get to the bottom of it. These folks were preying on sick people's desperation to end their suffering, and I was determined to find out what it was all about.

The more I searched, however, the more success stories I saw. There was even a video of an evening news report where a woman described how she had been in a wheelchair, and with the use of this drug not only did she get out of the wheelchair, but she was using absolutely nothing to aid her in walking.

I kept digging. I even tried researching on the well-known hoax websites, and found nothing negative.

I wanted to know everything about this drug and how I could get it. I found one website that listed a bunch of doctors who prescribe this medication, and a few "compounding" pharmacies (See Glossary) that actually make it. Yay! One of these pharmacies, Skip's Pharmacy, was a two-hour drive away from me, right here in Florida! I was so excited...I called!!

I almost had to laugh, because when a gentleman answered the phone and identified himself as "Dr. Phil", I was pretty much convinced at that point that it must have been a cruel joke.

I started asking this guy (Dr. Phil Giordano) a ton of questions about the drug; the first one being, "Is this a hoax?"

"Oh, no ma'm", he said, "This is no hoax. We distribute this drug to patients with Multiple Sclerosis all over the country."

"So," I asked, "How can I get this medication?"

After a few seconds, Dr. Phil gave me the name and telephone number of a doctor who prescribes the medication (it's all done over the telephone), and he assured me once again that this absolutely *was not* a joke, nor a hoax, but this was the real deal.

I thanked him and hung up the telephone. I was absolutely elated. I was determined to give this drug a try, but now I had to convince Dr. McRae. (Through my reading, I discovered that there are not a lot of physicians knew about this drug, nor did they approve of it. But why?)

I printed out a ton of research and faxed it over to Dr. McRae's office. I followed up with a telephone call, and asked the receptionist to please make sure the doctor got the information immediately. I took this opportunity to make another appointment with the doctor to discuss this medication, and my deteriorating condition.

I was still baffled as to why I had not heard of this medicine before. If it was providing all these benefits to all of these people, I wondered, why hadn't my doctor told me about it?

Chapter 12 – Be Bold!

My body was so sore and bruised from rotating the injection locations (See Glossary)...my hips, my thighs, upper arms, stomach...all one big bruise fest.

I had been taking injections since Thanksgiving, and here we were, six months later, and I was not getting any symptom relief. If anything, I was getting worse and experiencing more and more problems all the time.

In the midst of all of this going on, my new primary care doctor's office called to advise that my latest blood tests came back, and the T-cell count (See Glossary) was out of whack, so they made an appointment for me to see a Hematologist (See Glossary).

The Hematologist advised that my immune system (See Glossary) was extremely weak, so he wanted me to take some prescription medication which increases the number of white blood cells. He also wanted me to take a whole bunch of other supplements to get my immune system back to normal.

I knew in my gut this was happening because of the injections and steroids, and I wasn't really happy about the thought of taking more drugs. I mean, the MS medication is basically a chemotherapy drug, which kills the bad, as well as the good cells in your body. These are things doctors somehow "forget" to tell you when they are trying to convince you to take these drugs. For me, it was no surprise that my immune system was so weak.

That's it! I made my mind up that I was going to discontinue the injections, even if I couldn't get the LDN.

I informed the Hematologist of my thoughts about the drugs doing this to me, and explained that I didn't want to take any more treatments for anything. I was planning to stop the injections, and told him I was willing to bet any money that my immune system would return back to normal as soon as I did.

I may not have gone to medical school, but I knew my body. I refused to let all these doctors force me to take all of these toxic chemical treatments that were actually making me sick, with secondary problems popping up. What kind of quality of life was this for me?? I had so many years ahead of me, and I wasn't about to spend it holing myself up in my house, for fear of coming into contact with germs.

Well, as doctors do, he persisted in trying to convince me that I *needed* to follow his instructions in order to get better, but I refused. I was so exhausted and disgusted at this point, I just didn't want to hear about any more drugs!

To appease him, I accepted his prescriptions, but didn't have them filled.

I could hardly wait for my appointment with Dr. McRae. I planned to discontinue the injections and steroids so I could at least get my immune system back on track. I was very hopeful that after seeing the research I sent him, he was not going to hesitate in giving me the LDN.

Chapter 13 – I Don't Care!

Boy was I ever wrong! When Dr. McRae walked into the exam room, he was holding a stack of papers...my research papers! I thought, "Here we go! He's going to give me the LDN!"

I started to ask him if he looked over the research I had done. Just as the words were coming out of my mouth, he interrupted me and proceeded to throw the papers into the waste basket...right in front of my face!

"How rude", I thought! I was in shock, to say the least and let out a gasp of disbelief.

He took an abrasive tone, and proceeded to tell me he didn't support these "alternative treatments"; explaining that they are not proven, and there are no scholarly journals to back up any of the information I had given him.

So, "No", he didn't prescribe the LDN for me!

My excitement was quickly deflated. I pleaded with him to at least let me give it a try, just to see what it would do. I explained that I needed to get off of the injections. My health was not getting any better, and was having an everlasting relapse as we spoke. Besides, I reasoned, it couldn't be any worse than the current treatment I was injecting into my body.

He resisted me at every turn. He got very loud, and began citing his 12+ years in medical school, and his 20+ years in practice. He advised in no uncertain terms, that he knew what was best for me, and insisted he was *not* going to prescribe the LDN.

So, the obstacle standing between me and the possibility of good health was a stupid piece of paper? The lack of a scholarly journal was holding my good health hostage??? It's not like I was asking for street drugs or narcotics! This was an FDA-approved medication. Yes, it was approved for something other than MS, but doctors write prescriptions for "off-label" use of drugs all the time. For example, my sister (the one with MS) recently advised me that she had trouble staying awake during the day, so her doctor prescribed a drug for her which was originally FDA-approved to help people with Narcolepsy (a sleeping disorder).

As soon as I returned home that day, I pulled out the telephone number Dr. Phil had given me for Dr. Mulligan, the doctor who prescribed LDN. The woman who answered the telephone asked me several questions before faxing me some medical history forms to fill out. She also requested that I provide them with any transcripts from blood tests and MRI scans I had done. She further explained that after the doctor had an opportunity to review all of this information, they would call me to set up a telephone consultation. At that time, Dr. Mulligan would make a determination as to whether or not I was a good candidate to take the LDN.

In the meantime, I continued to suffer through these painful injections and take the awful immune system-killing steroids. By the way, neither one were doing anything to alleviate my symptoms. The only parts of my body that were *not* numb to some degree were my neck and head.

I could hardly wait to hear back from Dr. Mulligan's office.

Chapter 14 – The Search is Over

After my telephone consultation with Dr. Mulligan, I was elated that he was going to prescribe the LDN for me! It would be coming to me in the mail within a couple of days!

I could hardly contain my happiness. After reading about all the people whose lives were improved; I was very hopeful I was going to realize the same success.

Much to my delight, Dr. Mulligan also instructed me to stop giving myself the injections. He explained that the injections were "immuno-suppressants", and the LDN was and "immune-booster". The two do not work together. He *did* advise, however, that I needed to continue the course of steroids until they were gone. (Because of the tapering off process.)

So, for the next few days, I anxiously awaited my prescription of Low-Dose Naltrexone from Skip's Pharmacy. Had I been able to jump up and down for joy, I would have.

Two days after I spoke with Dr. Mulligan, I got home from work and checked my mailbox. There it was!!! My best hope for improved health, my LDN prescription.

I quickly tore the package open to examine the pills. They were little tiny capsules! I was so excited to be done with injections.

The instructions were to take one pill at bedtime, around 10:00 pm, because the medicine "works its magic" (See Glossary for an explanation of the mechanism of LDN) in the middle of the night while you're sleeping.

I had never been so excited to take medication in my life. So, here it was, 10 o'clock PM and I was just about to take my first dose. Tom went to bed, but I decided to stay awake, because I wanted to "see" what this pill was going to do to me. I wanted to be awake to witness this "miracle".

Chapter 15 – So Glad You're Back!

Be prepared to have your mind blown, because I tell you, mine certainly was! I kid you not when I say that very first dose of LDN changed my life!

I sat in the living room reading a book with the television on, in my efforts to stay awake. During this time, I kept putting my book down, consciously waiting for something to happen.

It is no exaggeration when I tell you, during the wee hours of the morning my hands slowly started tingling back to life. This amazed me! The very first dose! I was absolutely ecstatic. For months I couldn't even feel the fur on my cats when I pet them! Now, after a couple of hours, my fingers were "alive" again! This was absolutely crazy to me! I would not have believed it had I not experienced it for myself!

I was so excited, I wanted to scream. I limped into the bedroom as quickly as I could and woke Tom to tell him the good news! "It's working, it's working!"

Over the next couple of days, I carefully monitored my health. To my amazement, not only did the numbness throughout my whole body subside, but where I had been walking with a limp, dragging my right foot behind me, that went away too! My gait was just about back to normal! In addition, the tightness in my chest and torso from the MS Hug was gone! I also noticed I was no longer rushing to the bathroom for fear of losing my bladder. My dismal existence had almost completely turned around!

I know this all sounds really hard to believe, but every single bit of it is absolutely true. As I said, had I not experienced it for myself first hand, I would not have believed it. LDN really *was* a "miracle" drug, and I couldn't wait to add my success story to all of those I had seen on the Internet message boards just a few short weeks before.

Naturally, my excitement was mixed with disappointment. I couldn't help but be pissed off because Dr. McRae didn't want me to have this drug...the drug that literally erased months of my declining health.

Chapter 16 – Be Optimistic

The good news, my very next blood test came back completely normal. My immune system was 100% back on track. The even better news, my symptoms had almost completely disappeared.

After a few months, I went back to Dr. McRae to tell him (and show him) the good news. He looked at me skeptically and questioned as to how I was able to obtain the LDN. I explained the process of getting the medication, to which he just shook his head and rolled his eyes. (Disbelief or disapproval, I'm not sure which, but I didn't care. I was 100% better, no thanks to him.)

Although he was not responsible for giving me my life back, he agreed he would continue to order MRIs for me every six months.

So, months turned into years, four and a half, to be exact, with absolutely no relapses. Twice a year I went to Dr. McRae, and he would order my MRIs. Every time, they would call me to report no change in my films, and no active lesions; which meant no disease progression.

I firmly believed this was not a coincidence. I was convinced it was the LDN working to keep my symptoms under control. What other plausible explanation could there be?

Dr. McRae continued to perform regular exams on me, and asked about the LDN. He called it my "Voodoo Medicine". Surprisingly, although I had not relapsed in years, exhibiting absolutely no symptoms, it wasn't for his lack of trying to "scare" me into taking *his* drug of choice. He told me on several occasions that even though I hadn't been showing any visible symptoms, I could be "silently" relapsing, and getting worse under the surface. I reasoned to myself that for years my MRIs showed no new lesions and no disease progression; so I couldn't imagine his suggestion of "silent" deterioration was even remotely close to the truth!

Chapter 17 – The Cold, Hard Truth

Over the years, I have thoroughly researched all of the traditional "CRAB" drugs, as well as another mainstream treatment, the infusion of Tysabri (which I have never, ever heard anything good about!) In fact, I have heard very few stories of people realizing success using *any* of these traditional treatments.

I have seen the white papers and reviewed scholarly journals from new drugs as they come out. What I have read is astounding! Some people have actually died during clinical trials. (Something I'm sure your doctors won't tell you...mine didn't. He told me the new, "cutting edge" injectable drugs were what was best for me, because they "show promise". Besides, he defiantly advised, HE was the one who went to medical school!)

On the other hand, I have not heard of one single person who has experienced any adverse effects using LDN. What more proof do you need about the promise of continued health with this drug?
I've been taking it daily for over six years, which is a lot longer than some clinical trials even last! If LDN is not showing promise, I don't know what is! I am a walking billboard for this drug!

Chapter 18 – The Choice is Yours

There are fundamental differences between the traditional "approved" MS treatments and LDN. The first being, LDN is non-toxic. That's right, folks. LDN does not do the liver damage that the "normal", approved MS treatments do. Additionally, LDN *boosts* your immune system, where the approved drugs deplete it. The approved treatments are basically chemotherapy drugs (See Glossary), and they can't tell the good cells from the bad, so they just kill everything. This leaves you weak and exhausted and prone to viruses and serious infection.

By the way, in case you are reading this, and you or a loved one are injecting or infusing one of the "accepted" treatments, be sure to get regular blood tests to check your T-cell count and your liver enzymes (See Glossary). These are little details doctors tend to leave out during consults.

Chapter 19 – Lessons and Limitations Learned

It's six years later, and Dr. Mulligan continues to monitor my health on a regular basis...about once every three months. The conversation is always the same, no symptoms at all. My MRIs continue to stay the same; no new lesions, and no disease progression since 2007.

I'm not saying I don't have any struggles, because of the damage in my brain and spinal cord that *is* there that cannot be reversed. (Not yet, anyway!) Therefore, the muscles in my arms and legs are not as strong as they used to be.

The only time I feel weakness, discomfort, or have muscle spasms in my legs is if I get overheated or if I'm in weather where the temperature is less than maybe 45 degrees, or if conditions are windy. Once my body temperature is back to normal though, my symptoms go away. This is known as "Heat and Temperature Sensitivity" (See Glossary).

Through this journey, I am also learning my physical limitations. For example, I can't go running or jogging, because of the Clonus in my right leg. It causes my ankle stiffen up and not move properly. The doctor says I will always have it, and it will never get any better. I can't go hiking or do a lot of walking, especially in the heat. If I go to the gym, I can't overdo it, because if I get overheated, I start shaking and get physically ill.

I have never been one to tolerate being told I can't do something. But, through this process, you learn you are human, and it's very humbling. Sometimes I just physically cannot do things! I used to get very frustrated, but I have learned to accept it.

Chapter 20 – Be Loud!

I encounter people every day who are just like I was seven years ago, never having heard of LDN. I wished someone had approached me then about feeling better with this medication. It is because of this I make it a point to speak with anyone and everyone about this awful condition and the benefits I have found with LDN.

Although living with this disease is a very devastating thing to go through, it turns out I am a lot stronger than I ever imagined.

I have never been a person to take the hand I was dealt and just lie down and accept it. I also believe everything happens for a reason. I have a big mouth, and I was put on this Earth to use it to broaden the awareness of the benefits of LDN with regard to Multiple Sclerosis. People need to have some hope, and it's comforting to know there is something available that can possibly give them a better quality of life!

Because under normal circumstances I show no outward signs or symptoms, I am often met with reactions of disbelief when people find out I have Multiple Sclerosis. I almost feel guilty sometimes, because there are so many folks who DO show symptoms. (I'm getting the word out about LDN, but not fast enough, I suppose.)

I often walk right up to strangers in wheelchairs, sporting a cane, or getting around on a scooter, and I point blank ask them if they have been diagnosed with MS. I know it's very bold, and I realize some people want to keep their privacy. The way I see it, if I possess something that can help others, I'm going to make every attempt to do so. I want to share my good fortune with everyone. Why should I keep this "miracle" drug to myself? Would you?

It is my mission to change the landscape of the "accepted" treatments for Multiple Sclerosis and other chronic illnesses. If I can help just one person have a better quality of life, then my job is done!

Post Script

Wow! I wasn't prepared for the tears to come flowing out as I relived my story through the writing of this book. I can hardly believe I have gone through something so devastating (I was going downhill fast) but I got my life back! I am thriving!

As of the time of this writing, I have been made aware that a company called TNI BioTech, Inc. announced earlier this year that it has signed an agreement to acquire the "orphan" drug designation and patent rights for LDN.

In my opinion, this will likely make this medication more widely accepted in the medical community as a treatment for MS, and therefore more easily accessible to so many individuals suffering from chronic conditions who could benefit from this remarkable drug.

You can read more here at:

http://www.prnewswire.com/news-releases/tni-biotech-inc-acquires-the-exclusive-rights-to-low-dose-naltrexone-and-other-opioid-antagonists-for-the-treatment-of-inflammatory-and-ulcerative-diseases-of-the-bowel-186024712.html

Dr. Henry "Skip" Lenz, Pharm.D, owner of Skip's Pharmacy, a compounding pharmacy located in Boca Raton, Florida (where I personally have my LDN made for me) has joined TNI BioTech, Inc. as its Quality Control Officer. (Skip's Pharmacy has been the leading compounding pharmacy supplying LDN for over ten years.) You can read more here at:

http://www.tnibiotech.com/investor-relations/press-releases/135-dr-henry-skip-lenz-pharm-d-joins-tni-biotech-inc-as-quality-control-officer

It is interesting to note that I personally know three physicians, one a Gynecologist, and two General Practitioners, who have MS, and they all use LDN to keep their symptoms at bay.

My story doesn't end here, I'm afraid. Within a few years of my MS diagnosis, I started to experience symptoms of a whole different kind. You can read about it in my forthcoming book, **Thriving with Multiple Sclerosis and other Chronic Conditions.** You can start reading the first chapter by visiting this website:

www.TalkingBackToMS.com

https://www.facebook.com/groups/TalkingBackToMS/

Glossary:

As you read these definitions, please keep in mind that I am not a medical professional, and have done my best in trying to explain these terms in simple, basic terms.

<u>Multiple Sclerosis</u>: To put it into non-scientific terms, it is when you have damage to the protective coverings on nerve fibers in the brain and on the spinal cord. This interferes with the communication between the nerve fibers and the brain. Basically, it scrambles the signals, which is why sometimes you cannot move a particular limb, or you feel numb in certain areas. This is because there is damage to that part of the brain or spinal cord associated with the body part that is affected.

The name *Multiple Sclerosis* refers to multiple scars (or lesions or plaques) particularly in the white matter of the brain and spinal cord.

MS is thought to be caused when the body's own immune system attack and destroy the protective coverings on the nerves and nerve fibers, thus given the term "Auto-immune Disease". The risks of contracting this illness are dependent upon very complex and not well understood interaction of environmental as well as genetic factors. Studies continue in efforts to isolate these factors, and in recent years, there have been advances in medications used to suppress and slow down the progression of the disease.

Lumbar Plexus: A network of vessels and nerves of the lumbar region.

MRI: A test that uses magnetic fields and pulses of radio wave energy to create images of organs and other structures inside the body.

Clonus: This is a sign of some neurological conditions, such as Multiple Sclerosis, and is characterized by a series of involuntary contractions and relaxations of a muscle, most commonly at the ankle. In many cases it presents along with the condition of spasticity.

Lhermitte's Sign: This is an electrical sensation that runs down the back into your legs, most times when your head is bent forward.

Optic Neuritis: This is inflammation of the optic nerve in the eye, and may cause a partial, sometimes complete loss of vision, most commonly found in patients with Multiple Sclerosis.

Gadolinium: This is a chemical element injected into a subject during MRI testing as a contrast agent to indicate enhancement of scar tissue. (The FDA has warned that patients with diminished kidney function should avoid gadolinium-based contrast agents, as their kidneys are often unable to filter this chemical from their bloodstreams. A little known fact your doctor may not have told you.)

Brain Lesions: Also known as plaques, these are patches of inflammation in the central nervous system (CNS) in which the nerve cells have been stripped of their protective covering, or myelin.

Neurologist: This is a physician who is trained to investigate, diagnose, and treat disorders of the human nervous system.

Steroids: These are drugs which are used in efforts to reduce the severity and duration of relapses in patients with Multiple Sclerosis. Steroids are naturally occurring hormones in the human body. It is Glucocorticoids, which are steroids that occur naturally in the human body as cortisone and hydrocortisone, that are regularly prescribed to treat multiple sclerosis.

Steroids have a range of side effects, sometimes severe, since so many cells in the body have receptors for these glucocorticosteroids. Symptoms can include acne, depression, weight-gain, seizures, fatigue, and a condition known as adrenal insufficiency, where the adrenal glands (near the kidneys) do not produce enough of the chemicals they should which regulate organ function.

Lumbar Puncture: This test, also known as a spinal tap, requires a small amount of spinal fluid be extracted from the spinal column by inserting a needle between the vertebrae. The fluid is tested for the presence of an increased number of antibodies, known as "oligoclonal bands". These bands indicate increased immune system activity.

Although not specific to Multiple Sclerosis, this test is positive in a huge percentage of people with this illness.

FMLA: Stands for Family and Medical Leave Act. Under the United States Department of Labor Wage and Hour Division, FMLA entitles eligible employees of covered employers to take unpaid, job-protected leave for specified family and medical reasons. Eligible employees are entitled to twelve work weeks of leave in a 12-month period for a serious health condition that makes the employee unable to perform the essential functions of his or her job. See more at

http://www.dol.gov/whd/fmla/

<u>Oligoclonal Bands</u>: These are sometimes seen when a patient's spinal fluid is analyzed. These bands are an important indicator in the diagnosis of Multiple Sclerosis, as a large percentage of all patients with this illness have permanently observable oligoclonal bands. The bands are not specific to an MS diagnosis.

<u>"CRAB" Drugs</u>: This stands for Copaxone, Rebif, Avonex, and Betaseron, which are the four FDA-approved disease-modifying therapy drugs that are typically prescribed to slow the progression of Multiple Sclerosis. The medications are delivered via syringe either just under the skin, or directly into the muscle.

<u>Auto-Injector Pen</u>: This is a medical device designed for self-administration by patients to deliver a single dose of a particular drug.

<u>Evoked Potentials Tests</u>: These tests measure the time it takes for the nerves to respond to various forms of stimulation. There are several different types: Visual, where the eyes are stimulated by looking at a test pattern; Auditory, which is used to check when hearing is stimulated by listening to a test tone; and Somatosensory, which is when the nerves of the arms and legs are stimulated with an electrical pulse.

<u>Nerve Conduction Tests</u>: These tests measure how well and how fast nerves send electrical signals.

A needle attached to a recording machine by a wire is inserted into a muscle. The electrical activity is recorded while at rest and contracted.

Infusion Treatments – (Tysabri):– This drug is used as an alternative to the approved injectable medications, the CRAB drugs, and is administered by IV infusion about once every four weeks. Please read the official FDA information on this drug here:

http://www.drugs.com/pro/tysabri.html

MS "Hug": This abnormal sensation is caused by a lesion on the spinal cord, and is technically classified as "neuropathic pain". Like many symptoms, the "MS Hug" feels different for different people.

Generally felt all the way around the torso, it can be as low as the waist or as high as the chest; rarely as high as the shoulders. People often describe this feeling as being squeezed by a boa constrictor or wearing a tight girdle around their chest. Although it is very scary and uncomfortable, there is actually no danger of inhibiting one's ability to breathe.

Spasticity: Involuntary muscle contractions, usually caused by damage to the nerves that control those muscles. It most often affects the legs, and is very common for people with MS.

Foot Drop: This is the inability to lift the front part of the foot, causing the toes to drag the ground while walking. It is a symptom of an underlying neurological or muscular disorder. It can be temporary or permanent, depending on the cause.

Demyelinated Nerves: This is what happens when the protective cover (myelin sheath) on nerves is damaged. The mechanism of demyelination is not yet clearly understood, but it is thought that the body's immune system attacks itself (auto-immunity). When this damage occurs, it impairs the conduction of the signals in the affected nerves. This can cause a decrease in sensation (numbness), impaired movement, cognitive issues, and other problems depending on which nerves are affected.

Types or Stages of MS: There are four main very closely related stages (or subtypes) of Multiple Sclerosis:

> *Relapsing-Remitting (RRMS):* This stage is the most common form of MS. Most people will begin with this type. RRMS is characterized by the patient having an attack, or series of attacks (also called exacerbations), followed by times where there is complete or partial lessening of symptoms;
>
> *Secondary-Progressive (SPMS):* This is the second stage of RRMS. It is estimated that about 90% of those with RRMS will progress to this type.

Primary-Progressive (PPMS): This stage of the disease is most commonly found in men and is thought to occur in a very small percentage of those with MS. In this stage, the patient tends not to suffer from acute attacks, although the body gradually shows increased disability and impaired movement. Because the patient doesn't show signs of attacks, it is often difficult to diagnose this stage; and

Progressive-Relapsing (PRMS): This rare type of MS is characterized by starting out as progressive with very acute attacks, and having very little relief from accumulated symptoms. It is thought that less than 10% of patients with MS have this type.

There are several other types, not as widely known. They are:

Benign MS: This is a subtype of RRMS, and characterized by a person having a single attack, then the disease goes into remission for an extended period of time, in some cases, up to a decade or more. Patients with this form of MS may remain fully functional, although they may show evidence of brain or spinal cord atrophy upon MRI examination;

Malignant MS: (also called Acute MS or Marburg's Variant) This subtype is very serious, but very rare. In this stage, the disease progresses very quickly, and is most likely to cause significant disability within the first year of onset; and

Devic's Disease: (Also known as Neuromyelitis Optica "NMO") This is another (although rare) subtype of MS which is characterized by attacks to the spinal column and the optic nerves. It could result in blurred vision and pain in the eyes, and sometimes acute vision loss. The lesions are different than those of Multiple Sclerosis, although the two disorders are closely related.

Expanded Disability Status Scale (EDSS): This is a method used to quantify disability in Multiple Sclerosis patients. There are eight Functional Systems (FS) that are tested, which allow Neurologists to assign a score.

There are a lot of other scales, as well. I will list several here:

The Scripps Neurologic Rating Scale (SNRS)
The Krupp Fatigue Severity Scale (FSS)
The Incapacity Status Scale (ISS)
The Functional Independence Scale (FIM)
The Cambridge Multiple Sclerosis Basic Score (CAMBS)

The Functional Assessment of Multiple Sclerosis (FAMS)

You can read more about these disability scales at:

http://www.mult-sclerosis.org/expandeddisabilitystatusscale.html

Low-Dose Naltrexone (LDN): Naltrexone is a drug which was licensed by the FDA in 1984 for the treatment of opioid and alcohol addictions. On a basic level, at the full recommended dose, Naltrexone blocks a person's ability to "get high".

It has been prescribed at significantly lower doses as a treatment for a variety of diseases, including Multiple Sclerosis and other "auto-immune" diseases.

Clinical studies of this lower dose, "Low-Dose Naltrexone" (LDN) in the treatment of Multiple Sclerosis have been very limited.

Since 2010, however, there have been several studies and a pilot clinical trial involving 60 people with all types of MS. You can read more about these studies on the National MS Society web page.

http://www.nationalmssociety.org/about-multiple-sclerosis/what-we-know-about-ms/treatments/complementary--alternative-medicine/low-dose-naltrexone/index.aspx

(Personal note: This is very huge, because seven years ago, I could not find anything on their web page about LDN!)

Non-Toxic Drugs: Drugs that do not cause liver damage or dysfunction, such as Low-Dose Naltrexone.

Compounding Pharmacy: For the purposes of MS, and other chronic illnesses, since Naltrexone is currently manufactured as 50 mg tablets, a compounding pharmacist has to grind these into a powder and carefully measure the proper "Low-Dose" and put it into a capsule form.

T-Cells: These are the type of white blood cells that protect the body from infection. A low white blood cell count compromises your health and increases your chances of getting infectious diseases.

Rotating Injection Locations: When you receive a kit containing all the supplies you need to start injecting your CRAB drugs; there is a booklet included which diagrams all of the places on your body where you can inject your medications. It is recommended that you do not inject in the same place two times in a row. Typically, these locations are on the outer thigh, upper arm, hip, and stomach. Some patients develop injection site bruising and "dents" or depressions in the skin, due to loss of fat under the skin, known as "lipoatrophy".

Hematologist: This is a physician who specializes in blood conditions and disorders.

Immune System: The immune system is made up of organs, glands, and tissues that work together to protect the body from bacterial and viral infection.

LDN Mechanism while you sleep: It is recommended that LDN be taken between 8:00 and 10:00 PM, as the medication works while you sleep during the time of natural endorphin production (between 2:00 AM and 4:00 AM). Taking the LDN at bedtime causes a brief blockade of the opioid receptors, and subsequently produces a prolonged increase in endorphin production, boosting the immune system.

In people with diseases like Cancer and MS that are partially or largely caused by a deficiency of endorphins, restoration of the body's normal production of endorphins is the major therapeutic action of LDN.

Chemotherapy Drugs: Are used in the treatment of cancer, and contain one or more drugs that are toxic to the cells in the body (both good and bad). The intent behind the use of these drugs is to cure or prolong life. There are some chemotherapeutic drugs (a.k.a. the CRAB drugs) that have a role in the treatment of Multiple Sclerosis, and other "auto-immune" conditions.

Liver Enzymes: These are proteins present throughout the body, and they help speed up the routine and necessary chemical reactions in the body. Under normal circumstances, these enzymes are contained within the liver cells. If there is a problem with the liver, these enzymes will leak into the blood stream. Blood tests can assess the functions of the liver, and detect injury by determining the presence of these proteins in the blood.

Since your liver plays a key role in metabolizing medications, it is necessary, when taking certain prescription drugs, to have regular blood tests performed to check for liver damage.

Be very cautious, because some over-the-counter medications, such as Tylenol and Ibuprofen, can become toxic to the liver after extended periods of use.

(I recommend performing your own independent research on this subject.)

Heat and Temperature Sensitivity: In some cases, people with MS experience a temporary worsening of symptoms when the weather is hot or humid, they get overheated from exercise, or take hot baths or showers. These symptoms happen because the elevated temperature impairs the damaged nerve's ability to send the correct signals to the brain.

It is important to remember the symptoms are only temporary, and will normally subside as your body temperature normalizes.

You can read about this in more detail at the National MS Society website:

http://www.nationalmssociety.org/about-multiple-sclerosis/what-we-know-about-ms/treatments/exacerbations/heattemperatu re-sensitivity/index.aspx

Note: Obviously, these are not all the symptoms and signs associated with MS, but they are the ones I personally experienced from the time of my diagnosis, until I began taking the LDN.

About the Author:

Elizabeth J. Rhodes is not a medical professional, just a person who was diagnosed with Multiple Sclerosis who decided to defy the odds, and the doctors, and take her healthcare into her own hands. In doing so, she a treatment that enabled her to get her life back. She now spends a great deal of her time advocating for others who suffer from this, and other chronic and terminal conditions, in her efforts to raise awareness about the benefits of LDN. Her mission is to change the face of MS, and to share her good fortune with others who suffer from this sometimes debilitating illness.

www.TalkingBackToMS.com

https://www.facebook.com/groups/TalkingBackToMS/

www.ingramcontent.com/pod-product-compliance
Lightning Source LLC
Chambersburg PA
CBHW050425290526

45786CB00003B/1403